STEPPING STONES WITH CHILDREN: COUNSELLING GUIDE

Jovin F. Riziki and Sue Holden

T0166243

Acknowledgements

We express our deep appreciation to the people and organizations that have contributed to this guide. In Tanzania these include: Dr Theodor Tigawa from the Ministry of Health and Social Welfare; Dr Fausta Philip from the Muhimbili National Hospital; and Elisius Mkolokoti, Josephine Daffi, Rose Kadesha, and Martha Kamuhabwa of Pastoral Activities and Services for people with AIDS Dar es Salaam Archdiocese (PASADA). In the UK they are: Silvia Petretti of Positively UK; Dr Elspeth McAdam of the Taos Institute; Kate Holden of Time To Talk Counselling; and Gill Gordon and Alice Welbourn of the Salamander Trust.

About this counselling guide

We've written this guide for people who already have the knowledge, skills and experience needed to counsel adults about HIV and related issues. We haven't included basic information, such as what counselling is or key skills for counselling. Instead we've focussed on the *additional* knowledge and skills that counsellors need to work both with children who are affected by or living with HIV, and with their caregivers. We also outline the key steps to follow in different counselling situations involving children and caregivers.

This guide accompanies the *Stepping Stones with Children* manuals. Children and caregivers who attend *Stepping Stones with Children* workshops learn to appreciate their abilities, and to find ways of using these to improve their lives. For example: caregivers learn how to discipline children rather than hitting or otherwise punishing them, while children learn how to set boundaries regarding sexual intimacy, and how to protect themselves and others from sexual abuse.

> Counsellors can also benefit from doing *Stepping Stones with Children* exercises, both for their own self-knowledge and to understand better the issues their clients face. Throughout this guide – in boxes such as this – we highlight exercises in the *Stepping Stones with Children* manual which are particularly useful for counsellors to do themselves, or which contain useful information to inform their counselling. Ideally counsellors should go through the manual with a group of colleagues, to update their knowledge and familiarize themselves with the whole process.

Basics of counselling children

HIV counselling with children, as with adults, aims to help them cope with emotions and challenges relating to HIV and its effects, and to make informed choices that will improve their quality of life. Though the focus may be on HIV, counsellors need to see and work with the whole child: all the things that affect their life.

Counselling children includes:
✓ helping them tell their story;
✓ listening carefully;
✓ giving them correct and appropriate information;
✓ helping them make informed decisions;
✓ helping them recognize and build on their strengths;
✓ helping them develop a positive attitude to life.

Counselling children does not include:
✗ making decisions for them;
✗ judging or blaming them;

✗ interrogating or arguing with them;

✗ making promises you cannot keep;

✗ preaching to or lecturing them;

✗ imposing your own beliefs on them.

Our key tasks during counselling sessions with children and caregivers include:

- helping them understand their situation and how they are feeling by reflecting back what they have told us, both verbally and non-verbally;

- helping them explore their regrets and feelings of blame and anger;

- supporting them in seeing what they may be able to do to improve their situation, even though many factors are beyond their control;

- supporting them in making informed decisions;

- sharing useful information with them;

- supporting them in developing the courage and confidence to come up with their own strategies and hopes and plans for their future.

What's different about counselling children?

There are four key differences when counselling children as opposed to adults.

1. We must adjust what we say and do to suit the age and development stage of each child. There should be a big difference between the way we work with a five-year-old who may not yet be able to write, and a 15-year-old who may already be emotionally mature.

2. We usually work not with a single client, but with a child and their caregiver(s). We must attend to their different hopes and needs, and support them in working together.

3. We have to be willing and able to talk with children about sex and sexuality, and we may find this difficult.

4. We need to be mindful of local rules and laws regarding children, for example, knowing at what age and under what circumstances a child can get an HIV test without a caregiver's consent.

Below are some ideas about how to handle these four differences.

Adjusting the way we work to suit each child

Creating a friendly atmosphere

Children need to feel at ease if they are to communicate with us. Here are some things you can do to help create a friendly feel to your sessions.

- Smile!

- Wear a badge or necklace that is appealing to children.

- Have some toys and magazines available, appropriate to the age of the child.

- Tidy away paperwork and files.

- Put some appealing pictures or posters on the wall.

- Sit on the floor to play and chat with younger children.

Engaging with child clients

Many children are used to adults telling them what to do, criticizing them, and not listening. You need to do the opposite!

- Tell the child how long the session will last.
- Express your welcome, and let them know they can play and relax, e.g. 'Hello, you've come to play again!' or 'Great, it's time to chat with Joshua!'
- With young children, begin each session by playing together.
- With older children, start by chatting about something which interests them, such as sport, music, fashion or science.
- Give compliments and praise, e.g. 'You have put effort into that hair style' or 'You have done very well to get here in this rain! Thank you!'
- Don't hurry; listen carefully, and acknowledge what the child says.
- Use informal language, without jargon, in short sentences. Adjust what you say to suit the child's age and level of understanding.
- Be honest.
- Listen out for the child's abilities, and point them out, e.g. 'That was brave behaviour when you did that! You have the courage to do difficult things.'
- Be positive, e.g. speak of how we can live well with HIV, rather than framing HIV as a life-limiting illness.
- Provide information if it is needed, in a way the child can understand.
- Have suitable pictures or toys available, to help you explain ideas.
- Show interest in the child: each is unique.
- Be willing to engage with all topics and issues, not just those closely related to HIV.

Using different methods to help communication

When counselling adults we rely on talking to communicate. With children, we need some additional strategies. Often children may not know or be able to talk about their emotions. They may also hide their feelings because they do not want to upset their caregiver, or (in the case of abuse) get someone into trouble.

The following methods may be useful.

Drawing. Many children like to draw, and to be praised for their drawing. If you ask them to draw something related to what you want to explore, you can learn from what they draw and use it to help conversation. Don't make assumptions about their picture. Instead, use open questions to encourage them to talk: for example 'what's happening in this picture?' and 'how does this person feel about what's happening?'

If the child agrees, it may be useful for them to show their picture to their caregiver, for further discussion in a joint counselling session.

Storytelling. When a child finds it difficult to talk about painful issues, listening to a story about someone in a similar situation can be very comforting. It can give them a sense of being understood, and help them recognize that they are not alone.

A story can also serve as a tool for problem solving around the child's own situation. Tales of characters who overcome difficulties in their lives help children imagine overcoming their own difficulties.

If you use storytelling, avoid using real names or events. At the end of the story encourage the child to talk about what happened, so you know if they have understood it. You can then explore the relevance of the story to their own life.

Note that you don't have to be the storyteller. You can help children make up their own stories, based on a topic that you give them, for example, 'Tell me a story about a little girl who was ill but then got better.'

Play. Having toys available for children to play with – such as a few boxes and animal or human figures – allows them to relax. You may want to shape their play through a request such as 'show me a happy day in your family'. Observing their game and asking open questions should help you understand their emotions, and may reveal needs and problems. You could also use their game to explore options, e.g. 'what would happen if that character doesn't want to go to the clinic?'

Writing about experiences. Older children may like to write poems, fictional stories, or accounts of their own experiences, which you can then discuss together. Be sure that the child is happy to write; for some, such 'school work' might put them off coming to counselling sessions.

> If the people you are counselling have been to *Stepping Stones with Children* workshops, you can use some of those concepts in your sessions, such as the idea of getting back 'on our hub' when we are feeling distressed (see Session 2). You could also remind the children about the breathing exercises, and do them together.

Working with children and their caregivers

Sometimes, and if allowed, you will counsel an older child who lacks the support of a caregiver, does not want their caregiver to attend, or whose caregiver will not or cannot attend. In such cases you will have one-to-one sessions with the child, adjusting how you work to suit them. If the child lacks any adult carer in their life, it will be particularly important to link them to support networks.

Mostly, however, children come to counselling with a caregiver. Or, if you are visiting them at home, there may be other family members around. You may want to work with the child and caregiver separately (if allowed), or together, or both. You will need to use your judgement to decide what is best, depending on the personalities and situation in each case. We give some general suggestions below.

When to work with a child and without the caregiver

You may want to work with a child outside the caregiver's presence if:
- you want to create a trusting relationship with the child, without the distraction of the caregiver's presence;
- you want to explore issues and feelings with the child that they are unlikely to want to discuss in front of the caregiver, e.g. how the child feels about the caregiver, whether the child is abused, and other personal topics (such as their sexual life);
- the caregiver tends to interfere with the child's communication, e.g. talking on behalf of the child, or taking over the child's game;

- the caregiver's presence seems to inhibit the child from communicating with you, e.g. the child looks to the caregiver for permission to speak, and seems to say what they are 'allowed' to say, rather than what they would like to say.

Depending on the rules in your country and organization, you may need to have another adult present (e.g. a nurse) while the caregiver is not in the room.

When to work with a caregiver and without the child

You may want to work with a caregiver outside the child's presence if:
- you want to explore certain issues and feelings with the caregiver, e.g. their fears about the child, or other topics about which the adult will not speak truthfully within the child's hearing;
- the child is distracting, e.g. interrupting, needing attention.

When to work with the child and caregiver together

You may want to work with both the child and caregiver at once:
- when you want to facilitate discussion and problem-solving between them;
- when you want to share the same information with both child and caregiver;
- when a child is afraid of, or uncomfortable, being alone with you.

Tips

- When working alone with the child or the caregiver, you can give the other person a useful task to do while they are waiting. For example, ask them to draw a picture, make up a story, write about how they feel, create a mind map, or read some information. You can then explore what they have produced or learned when you meet with them later.
- If a caregiver is reluctant to let you speak with the child alone, explain that it is normal and useful to give children some one-to-one time with a counsellor. Politely and assertively request that they allow the child to take this opportunity. If they still refuse, explore why. What are they afraid of? Perhaps it would help if there were another adult in the room? Explain that there are issues you want to explore with the child, for their benefit, and that you will update the caregiver afterwards.
- When working alone with a child, make sure the child knows where their caregiver is, and how long the one-to-one part of the session will be.

Counselling children about sexuality

As counsellors, we are used to discussing sexual issues with adults but we may struggle to do so with children. Here are some points for you to consider, to improve your ability to counsel children about sexuality.

Be aware of your own opinions and beliefs, and be able to put them aside. No child should feel judged by you, for example, if they tell you they have done something you feel is morally wrong, such as having sex or feeling attracted to someone of the same sex as them.

Remember that sex and sexuality are not 'adult issues'. Our cultures may discourage us from talking to children about sex and sexuality, but all humans are sexual beings. Talking with children about sex does not lead to them having sex, but it does make them better informed to make better decisions.

Reduce embarrassment. Find and practise saying age-appropriate words and phrases to use when counselling children about sexuality. Also, be prepared to use the vocabulary that they use. Clients will be less inhibited and embarrassed if you are calm and confident.

Have your own support system. Ensure you can get the professional support of your supervisor or mentor to help you cope, confidentially, with emotional issues that may arise, e.g. when counselling a child who is being abused.

> Session 21 is all about children's sexual feelings and sexual safety. It will help you to talk about such issues with them.

Following local rules and laws regarding children

Written laws vary from country to country, as does the way in which rules are interpreted in practice. Your organization should have written protocols to guide its counsellors, setting out the key rules and practices, such as the following.

Consent

- age at which children need parental consent to have HIV counselling, and to have an HIV test;
- rules on how you explain the issue of consent to children and caregivers, and how you assess whether consent has been given or withheld;
- exceptions to the rules on parental consent, e.g. for homeless children, those who have been sexually assaulted, and 'mature minors'.

Confidentiality

- laws relating to confidentiality, and procedures to ensure confidentiality;
- rules on how to discuss and make agreements about confidentiality with children and their caregivers;
- rules on children's right to know their HIV status versus caregivers' wish to withhold test results from them;
- exceptions to rules on confidentiality, e.g. that it will be broken in a medical emergency if health workers need to know what medication the child is taking.

Unlawful sex and abuse

- age at which children can legally have heterosexual sex;
- laws relating to homosexual sex;
- laws and procedures to follow regarding abuse;
- laws relating to the sexual transmission of HIV.

Confidentiality and ethics

This section gives an overview of what we, when counselling children, need to do regarding confidentiality and ethics.

Confidentiality

We all have the right to confidentiality. Working as HIV counsellors, there is a danger that we become relaxed about it, assuming that our client's status is widely known because they come for our HIV services. We must not fall into that trap. At every stage we need to be aware of maintaining confidentiality, and discussing it with caregivers and children. This includes:

- explaining that what we discuss in counselling sessions is confidential, and that we will only share information with others with the client's consent;

- setting out who will know the results of the HIV test within the health setting;

- explaining situations when we will break confidentiality, for example, if the law says we must report sexual abuse, or if we will take action when we believe that the life of the child or another person is at risk;

- supporting the caregiver and child in exploring the pros and cons of disclosing their HIV status to others;

- respecting the decision of those children and caregivers who do not want to disclose their HIV status to others;

- if appropriate, supporting the child and caregiver in disclosing their HIV status when they feel ready, enlarging their circle of shared confidentiality;

- if working in a support group, setting norms to maintain a shared confidentiality understood and adhered to by all the participants.

Ethical protocols when counselling children and their caregivers

- Explain that your role is to listen, ask questions, and help the child and caregiver make sense of their situation. You may give information and might make suggestions, but you will not advise or tell them what to do.

- Ensure that each session is a place of safety for the child, free from interruptions. State when the session will finish, and stick to that boundary.

- Explain and maintain confidentiality (as above).

- If you need to break confidentiality, first inform the child and caregiver. Discuss this with them and try to involve them in the decision-making.

- Refer children or caregivers who are in your social or professional network (e.g. your daughter's friend) to a different counsellor.

- Know your own limits. Refer cases to a peer or senior colleague if more expertise is needed for the benefit of the child.

- Maintain a professional distance. This includes not making any inappropriate physical contact and managing your emotional involvement so that it is in your control, and does not affect your ability to counsel the family.

- Use sessions with your supervisor or mentor to reflect on your practice, and (while maintaining confidentiality) to discuss ethical dilemmas and other difficulties that arise in your work.

- Ensure the client's identity is protected if their case is used professionally, e.g. in research or a presentation. It is good practice to change geographical location as well as names.

Counselling children for HIV testing

We assume that if you are working as a counsellor for HIV testing, you have had yourself tested for HIV. You were willing to put yourself through the process, and you know how it felt for you. If you have not yet taken an HIV test, please do so before counselling others about it.

The golden rules for HIV testing are that it is voluntary, confidential and carried out with informed consent. Applying these rules is a little different in the case of children than with adults.

Voluntary. Neither the adult or child is being forced to take the test.

Confidential. The usual protocols apply about keeping the results confidential, but in many countries a child's results may be given to a caregiver and withheld from the child. In other words, they are kept confidential from the child. One part of the pre-testing process is to support the caregiver in deciding how to manage sharing the results with the child.

With informed consent. Usually it will be the caregiver who needs to give informed consent. This means understanding the risks and benefits, and actually choosing to have the test, not just agreeing with a health worker's suggestion. Once we have the caregiver's informed consent, we must then seek the child's assent (agreement) to go ahead with the test. If the child disagrees then the test cannot be carried out, as it would not be voluntary.

In some cases, when an older child attends without a caregiver, it is allowable to get informed consent from the child. Depending on the rules where you work, such cases might include situations of rape, pregnancy and possible accidental exposure to HIV.

Pre-test counselling

Below we outline key steps to take when a caregiver and child come to you for pre-test counselling. We suggest different ways of handling children by age, but you should be guided by their knowledge and maturity in addition to their age. We note that for babies and infants the process is undertaken with the caregiver, and there is little or no need for the child's involvement.

HIV testing should be carried out primarily for the child's own benefit. For example, if a child is sickly and not getting better, and Anti-Retroviral (ARV) treatment is locally available for people who need it, then a test would probably be to the child's benefit, to discover whether or not HIV is the cause of their ill health. Or, if a child may have been exposed to HIV, and wants to know their status, then testing is in their interest provided they have the emotional maturity and support to cope with the result and its repercussions. There is a risk, though, that we or caregivers may want to get a child tested because of our own fears and anxieties, rather than thinking first of the child. So we need to reflect on our own feelings, and take care to explore each caregiver's motivation for getting a child tested.

Reasons why you might not test a child after pre-test counselling include:

- significant emotional distress, i.e. the caregiver or child cannot participate meaningfully in the session, and would be unlikely to cope with a positive result;
- imminent risk to the safety of the child, because the child or caregiver has stated that a positive result is likely to provoke a harsh response from a family member;

> The *Stepping Stones with Children* workshops address these issues, enabling children and caregivers to understand and accept HIV, and to create a more positive environment for those affected by HIV.

- the child lacks the social support to assist them in coping with a positive result and its implications;
- the child does not give their assent to the test.

Pre-test counselling for caregiver and child

Working first with the caregiver alone
Explain that what you discuss together is confidential, and how and when there might be exceptions to this.
Discuss why they want the child to be tested for HIV. Find out if the child may have been exposed to HIV.
Get a sense of how much the caregiver knows about HIV and AIDS, and correct any misconceptions. What have they told the child, and how much do they want the child to know?
Discuss and explain the benefits and challenges of knowing the child's HIV status.
Explore ways of involving the child in the decision to have a test, and in finding out the results. Look at the pros and cons of more or less involvement, and try to find a balance. Explain that, in most cases, children benefit from having information, as long as it is accompanied by support.
Discuss how a positive HIV result will affect the caregiver and child. Also discuss how a negative HIV result will affect them (e.g. it might make the child feel guilty if a sibling has HIV).
If it seems that testing would benefit the child, and the caregiver wants to proceed with the test, invite the child into the session. If the benefit to the child is in doubt, do not proceed; instead, suggest another meeting to review the child's health in six months' time. If the caregiver does not want to proceed, and the child may have been exposed to HIV, invite them to come for another pre-test session within the next few months.

Working with the child and caregiver together		
For children aged 3 to 5	**For children aged 6 to 12**	**For over 12s**
Smile and help the child feel at ease by playing or chatting.		
Explain that what you discuss together is confidential, and exceptions to this.		
Let the caregiver discuss their concerns with the child and encourage the child to respond.	Let the caregiver discuss their concerns with the child, and encourage discussion between them.	
Find out what the child knows about why they are there. Correct any misconceptions.		Find out what the child knows about why they are there, and what they know about HIV and AIDS. Correct any misconceptions. If the child seems inhibited, suggest that the caregiver leaves the session.

Working with the child and caregiver together		
For children aged 3 to 5	**For children aged 6 to 12**	**For over 12s**
If necessary, explain with appropriate language, e.g. 'Did you know that germs can get in people's blood? Luckily, if we know a germ is there, and it is making a person feel sick, we can use medicine to control it. Then the person can stay healthy. So it's good to know if the germ is there or not. If we take a little bit of blood from you we can find out if you have a certain germ.'	If necessary, explain with appropriate language, speaking either about 'a germ', 'a virus', or HIV, according to how much the child knows and what you have agreed with the caregiver. Explain the benefits and challenges of knowing if there is something in their blood.	If necessary, explain about HIV and HIV testing and the benefits and challenges of knowing your own HIV status.
Explain how the blood is taken, how long it takes to test it, and what the possible results mean.		
Discuss how the results would be shared, who would support the child if they have HIV and, in this case, how they would get care and treatment when needed.		
Ask if the child has any questions or concerns, including about the disadvantages of having an HIV test. Give honest answers they can understand.		
Ask the child 'shall we find out if the germ is in your blood?'	Ask the child 'shall we find out if there's anything in your blood?'	Ask the child 'shall we find out if HIV is in your blood?'
If the child assents (agrees), seek consent from the caregiver. Stress that it's important to come back for the results. If the child disagrees, invite them back for another session.		
If relevant, explain about, or refer clients to, other services, e.g. sexual and reproductive health services.		

Pre-test counselling for children attending alone

In cases where a child attends pre-test counselling alone, you will need to assess if they are able to give informed consent to have an HIV test, in terms of both local laws and their emotional maturity. To give informed consent, the child must:

- understand the possible risks and benefits of testing;
- be willing to accept support in coping with the test result, especially if it is positive.

If they are legally and emotionally able to give consent, then follow the same steps as for working with a caregiver. Ask if they can think of someone who will support them in case the result is positive, and who can accompany them to the post-test counselling.

If the child cannot legally give informed consent, follow the same steps, but explain that to access the test, if they still want it, they will need to return with a caregiver. If the child is reluctant to bring their primary caregiver, explore why. Perhaps you can help by meeting with and supporting the caregiver. Alternatively, explore whether the child has someone else in their support network who can take on the role of caregiver. If so, when meeting that person you must explain why they have been asked to take on the role, and they must agree to observe confidentiality.

If you feel the child cannot give consent owing to lack of understanding or willingness to accept support, ask them to come back for another session in which you can talk about it further.

Post-test counselling

Post-test counselling helps caregivers and children to understand the test result and its implications, and to consider and plan for what will happen next.

How you run each post-test session will depend on what you agreed with the caregiver and child in the pre-test session and their thoughts in the post-test session. For example, you may have agreed that the child gets their results from you without their caregiver present, that they both hear the result at the same time from you, or that the caregiver shares the result at home, when the time is right.

Here is a general outline for you to adapt. It is for the situation in which you first tell the caregiver, and then bring the child into the session to hear the result.

Working first with the caregiver alone	
Check that they know why they have come, and that they are ready to receive the result.	
Give the result and explain what it means. Be sure that they understand.	
Give time for reflection, to consider how they feel about the result.	
For a negative result	*For a positive result*
Check they understand how HIV is transmitted, and discuss how to reduce the child's likelihood of acquiring HIV.	Discuss the next steps in terms of referral and counselling. Emphasize the availability of care and support, and – when needed – effective treatment to enable the child to live well and have their own children without HIV.
If relevant*, explain about the window period and the need for another test.	Review ways of staying healthy and avoiding onward transmission, and address any fears the caregiver has.
Discuss how to share the result with the child, who will do this, and when.	
	Discuss disclosing the result to others; emphasize that there is no hurry, you can talk about this further in future sessions.
Working with the child and caregiver together	
If appropriate, invite the child into the session. Find out how they are feeling, and check if they are ready to receive the result.	
Give the result, using the same terms you used in the pre-test session, or let the caregiver give the result.	
Check that the child has understood the result, and give them time to ask questions and raise concerns.	
If relevant*, explain about the window period and the need for another test.	Emphasize that with treatment, care and support, people can live long and healthy lives with HIV: 'We will work together so that you cope with this and live well.' Reassure them that children with HIV can grow up to have their own babies who do not have HIV.

Discuss with the child things they can do to keep HIV out of their blood.	Discuss how they feel about disclosure. Explain that telling others can be useful, but can also cause problems when other people don't know enough about HIV. There's no hurry; it's something to talk about more in future sessions.
	Reassure them that they are not alone – there are other children in the same situation. Arrange for referral to a peer support group, if they would like, and follow-up, and check that the caregiver and child understand the next steps.

If your session is with an older child (who gave informed consent) with no caregiver present, then follow the first half of the steps above. Be sure to give them time to express themselves, and to discuss their fears. If the child doesn't feel ready to receive the result, or lacks the support or emotional stability to cope with it, make a plan to enable them to become ready, and to return for another session.

In the case of an unclear (indeterminate) result, follow the same process but explain that the result was not clear, and that the test will need to be done again in two weeks' time. Emphasize that we do not yet know the child's HIV status. The unclear result could be due to a problem in the labs, or because the child is in an early stage of having HIV, when it is easy to pass HIV to someone else. So it's important to avoid any possibility of transmission. This additional period of uncertainty is likely to be stressful for your clients, so give them time to talk about their concerns, and encouragement to come back for the re-test.

* If a child has an HIV-negative result, when should we re-test?

WHO advice is to re-test people who: are pregnant; have an ongoing risk of exposure to HIV (including breastfeeding from someone who has HIV); or have experienced a specific incident of HIV exposure in the past three months.

Children may also want to re-test owing to anxiety. If reassurance and exploring their fears does not work, re-testing may reduce their anxiety.

Disclosure of HIV status sometime after HIV testing

It is quite usual for caregivers to have a child tested for HIV, find that the child does have HIV, but not pass that information on to the child. Equally, caregivers may not disclose their own HIV-positive status to their children. There are many reasons for keeping quiet. In general, though, it is better for the child to know their own and their caregivers' HIV status, particularly as they get older, provided they are supported to understand and cope with the situation and to live positively.

Box 1 Case study: Disclosing to a child sometime after HIV testing

In one *Stepping Stones with Children* workshop a 10-year-old boy with HIV, who did not know his status, said 'If I had HIV I would want to kill myself.' The session on HIV was a few days later. All the children and caregivers learned about the differences between HIV and AIDS, and how treatment can keep those people who need it to stay healthy and live happy and productive lives. Some days after that, the boy's caregiver told the boy that he had HIV. His immediate response was 'Do I have HIV or do I have AIDS?' She replied, 'You have HIV because you are taking your treatment very well and that is keeping the HIV from making you feel sick. So you are doing so well.' The boy replied 'That's OK then', and went off happily to play football with his friends. The caregiver was delighted and very relieved to have shared this secret with the boy.

There are several situations in which you may play an important role, facilitating disclosure of a caregiver's or child's HIV status to a child:

- A caregiver might approach you for help, thinking that they want to tell the child or that the child wants to know, but feeling unsure how to do it.

- A child might, when attending clinic for tests and treatment, ask why they are having to take medication. The health worker would not be able to tell them straight out – this would be too sudden, and it would be without the caregiver's cooperation – but as part of their duty of care to the child they should enable the child to get an answer. In this situation the health worker would ask the caregiver to meet with a counsellor to discuss disclosure.

- A health worker might want the child to know their own status because it is likely to help them. Disclosure can help in several ways: the knowledge reduces stress and anxiety for children who suspect their status, or that of their caregiver; it enables the child to get the support of peers; and having full information can help those on treatment to adhere to it better. However, the health worker or counsellor must never impose their views on those in their care.

We must also be aware of the possible disadvantages of disclosure to children. These include the child becoming depressed, and being angry and resentful, both about their status and the fact that it has been withheld from them. There is also the risk that the child experiences stigma and discrimination as a result of disclosing to others.

Session 13 is all about HIV testing and talking about HIV with children. It contains some useful resources for counsellors, including on fears and benefits relating to sharing an HIV diagnosis with children, and help for caregivers on how to tell their children.

Be sure to know the rules in your country and the policies in your organization about disclosure to children. For example, in some countries health workers are not allowed to talk with children about their HIV status without the caregiver's consent, with the exception of children who are sexually active, pregnant or married. However, these rules go against the rights of the children to have information about their own health. As counsellors, our role is to work with caregivers to find the best solution in their situation. Here are some key steps to follow.

Establish what the caregiver has told the child about their health and HIV status.
Explore the caregiver's thoughts and feelings about the situation.
Explore the possible benefits and disadvantages of disclosing to the child (see Exercise 13.6, for a good summary).

Explore the possible advantages of *not* disclosing to the child (e.g. the child may feel less anxious) and the possible disadvantages (e.g. they might find out accidentally from someone else). This might take several sessions; the caregiver should feel in charge, and not under pressure.

Caregiver decides not to disclose	Caregiver cannot decide	Caregiver decides to disclose
Respect their decision.	Invite them to come for another session.	Support them in planning how to do it (see Exercise 13.7). This might include practising disclosure through role play.
Encourage them to think about it again in the future, as the child grows up and the situation changes.	Link them to a support group where they can meet other caregivers and find out about their experiences.	Invite the caregiver and child back for follow-up sessions.

Supportive counselling for children living with HIV and their caregivers

The ultimate aim of ongoing HIV counselling is to support children living with HIV to cope and live well.

In reacting to their HIV status, children and caregivers are likely to go through the five recognized stages of dealing with grief and loss. These are: denial, bargaining, anger, despair, and acceptance. Note, they may not go through the stages in that order, and may repeat stages. This is normal and there is no fixed pattern. As a counsellor your aim is to support the child and caregiver in reaching the point of acceptance, in order that they can live well with HIV.

Just after disclosure

This is when your involvement will be most intensive. Ideally you will book follow-up sessions with the child and caregiver, particularly if their reaction indicates that they need or want support.

At this stage it is very important to address and resolve possible issues of anger and blame, which may be felt by both the caregiver and the child. Try to ensure that the child has someone they can talk to in addition to you, e.g. a caregiver, other relative, or friend, whom you might identify before disclosure. You can also tell them about support groups they can attend.

Ongoing counselling

Through your ongoing support to the child and, if relevant, caregiver, you aim to:
- help them accept the reality of living with HIV;
- explore and deal with their fears and concerns;
- ensure they understand that it is *noone's fault* that they have HIV;
- support them in considering whether they wish to disclose their HIV status to others and, if so, to whom, and how to do it;
- tell them about peer support options, if locally available;
- provide appropriate information about HIV and other issues as they arise, such as sexual health;

> Exercise 14.3 helps caregivers deal with their fears about transmitting or acquiring HIV.

- connect the child to available support services – medical, psychological, social and spiritual – to widen their sources of support;
- support the child in understanding treatment – when they need it, how it supports their health, and why taking medications regularly is important – so they can live well with HIV;
- help the child develop their self-esteem, a positive attitude towards life, and their hopes and plans for the future.

When providing supportive counselling you should:
- work with a positive attitude and show optimism and reassurance;
- acknowledge that the child is undergoing a traumatic experience;
- try to ensure that the child gets holistic care;
- create a safe and confidential environment;
- if possible, work with a caregiver who acts as a secure base for the child;
- seek help whenever the need arises.

Counselling children on specific issues

Confidentiality and disclosure

As part of our usual practice, we make sure that clients understand the rules we and other colleagues follow regarding confidentiality. We also set out the situations in which we will break confidentiality. In addition to this, we need to support children in considering how they manage information about their own HIV status. Here are some key points that children need to consider, with your facilitation.
- It can help us to live well with HIV if we can think of a trusted adult or a close friend whom we can tell. Then we have someone to talk to about HIV when we are feeling concerned. Telling someone you have HIV is called 'disclosure'.
- The first steps towards disclosure are that we need to know the facts about HIV, and understand what it is and what it isn't.
- Sometimes we may decide not to tell others. This is not because there is anything wrong with having HIV; we do not keep this information to ourselves because we are ashamed. It is because other people may not yet have the right information or understanding about HIV and AIDS. If they don't understand it properly they may react badly, in ways which can hurt us.
- Once you have told other people, you cannot undo having told them. Also, you cannot know what the repercussions will be. They may be positive or negative, or both.
- You may not need to maintain 100 per cent secrecy. It's possible to develop 'shared confidentiality'; this means sharing your status with people that you trust, who will not tell anyone else without your permission. The *Stepping Stones with Children* workshops create a community of people who do understand about living with HIV, and who can support each other.
- Many people find that joining a peer support group of other adults or children is useful, as you can then talk with people who are experiencing the same issues.

Counselling about Anti-Retroviral Therapy

It is important to explain to caregivers that the first way to treat anyone with HIV, including children, is to give them love, care and support, nutritious food, safe housing and, where possible, exercise. These are the basic building blocks of good health. Medication works most effectively when these foundations are in place.

Supporting children and caregivers in accessing and sticking to treatment, when their bodies need it, is a key part of ongoing counselling. You'll need to:

- share information with clients about where they can get HIV medication (Anti-Retroviral medication, or ARVs), how this works, and the importance of monitoring its effect on our bodies;
- support them in making ARVs part of their daily routine by linking the act of taking them to daily tasks such as brushing teeth, putting clothes on, or having dinner;
- use simple and non-scary ways of explaining how HIV affects the body and the immune system and how ARVs help people with HIV to stay healthy, e.g. 'the immune system is like a team of farmers which gets rid of weeds so that the crops grow well. HIV tries to stop the farmers from weeding, but treatment lets them get on with it ...';
- encourage and support children in taking their ARVs regularly: explain that not taking ARVs regularly leads to illness, and that the HIV in our bodies can become resistant to the medication;
- assess whether clients have been taking ARVs regularly by using their feedback, medication counts, and biological markers such as their CD4 and viral load count;

> Read Exercise 14.7 to learn from children living with HIV about what helped them take their medication regularly.

- explore with children and caregivers any problems they may have with taking ARVs regularly, including treatment toxicity and side effects, and support them in developing strategies to deal with such problems;
- refer issues that arise in the health setting (e.g. unfriendly staff, or demands for bribes) to the relevant authority.

Counselling abused children

In general, abused children are likely to behave differently from children who are not abused. You may observe, for example, a child who is particularly withdrawn, who does not make eye contact, and who is unable to talk about their feelings. Here are the main forms of child abuse and the signs to look out for.

Type of child abuse	Signs of abuse
Neglect is failure to provide food, clothing, shelter, medical care and supervision to the extent that the household can afford to do so.	• child is dirty, has inadequate clothes • stunted growth • existence of treatable health problems • not in school
Physical abuse involves aggression directed at the child. > Table 9.1 sets out the difference between punishing children (e.g. beating them) and using positive discipline; this may help you when counselling caregivers who use physical punishment.	• cuts, burns, bruises and fractures • child is harmed by more 'accidents' than is usual • fear of a particular person or object

Type of child abuse	Signs of abuse
Emotional abuse includes excessive criticism, name-calling, ridicule, destruction of personal belongings, humiliation, and withholding of communication and love.	• anxiety • low self-esteem • depression • disassociation (detachment from reality) • drug and/or alcohol use • anger • self-harming (e.g. cuts to arms) • early sex and casual sex
Sexual abuse includes indecent exposure of genitals, showing pornography to a child, creating pornography involving a child, sexual touching, sexual intercourse, and selling the sexual services of children. Exercise 26.3 compares caring and sexual touches, which may help you explore and assess whether a child is being abused.	• temper, irritability and crying • fear of a particular person or object • disrespectful behaviour • nightmares and bed wetting or soiling • greater orientation to sexuality issues than expected for their age • genital or anal pain, bleeding or itching • difficulties in walking or sitting • pregnancy

Note that the presence of these signs does not prove that the child is being abused; an anxious and withdrawn child may simply be shy and badly affected by problems in their life, such as the loss of their parent(s). However, the presence of signs does mean that you should look a little closer.

If you suspect that a child is being abused you could:
- explore the issue with the child when the caregiver is not present:
  - ask gentle questions, or explore using a story or game, but do not challenge the child or try to force them to speak about it;
  - convey that when a child is abused (e.g. the child in a story you tell) it is never their fault; it is up to adults to protect children;
  - explain that when adults fail to protect a child then something needs to change; reassure them (e.g. through your story) that action can be taken, abuse can be stopped, and the child's life can improve;
- explore your concerns with the caregiver when the child is not present;
- explore the issue with both child and caregiver if the caregiver is not the person doing the abuse.

Exercise 26.4 includes ideas about what children can do to protect themselves from sexual abuse, and what caregivers can do to prevent it.

You could use Exercise 26.5 to support a child in practising different ways they might respond to sexual approaches.

If a child tells you that they are being abused you should believe them; children rarely lie about abuse, particularly sexual abuse (bear in mind that abusers often tell children that there's no point in telling anyone as no one will believe them). You should not show shock, but can respond with the following key messages:

1. I trust you.

2. I appreciate that you have told me.

3. I am sorry that this has happened to you.

4. It is not your fault that this has happened to you.

5. I need to know more so that I know the best way to help you.

Talk to the child about who else will need to be told (e.g. if you are legally obliged to report the abuse) and who else they think needs to know. Explain clearly what needs to happen next, as a result of the abuse, and what kinds of protection and support are available.

If the child is willing for you to discuss the issue with the caregiver, bring them into the session and facilitate a discussion between the child and caregiver about what to do next.
- If the police are to be involved you may need to refer the child for a medical examination (with the caregiver's consent) for evidence of physical or sexual abuse.
- If appropriate, and with the caregiver's consent, arrange for post-exposure prophylaxis (also known as PEP, to reduce the risk of acquiring HIV) and emergency contraception for the child, as well as testing and treatment for sexually transmitted infections, including HIV.

If the caregiver or their partner is the perpetrator of the abuse you will need to support the child in considering what to do. You may need to report the abuse. If possible, bring a different adult, whom the child trusts, into the conversation. Your aim is to support the child in reaching a situation where the abuse no longer happens, or they can avoid it, or it is reduced. Be aware that the abuse could increase if the perpetrator is challenged and the child is not given protection from them.

Counselling children on death and dying

Sometimes as counsellors we must support children in coping with the death or approaching death of a parent, sibling or friend, or with their own death. We need to help them understand death as a fact of life, and to support them through the stages of dealing with grief and loss: denial, bargaining, anger, despair, and acceptance.

Counselling about death and dying may cause us anxiety due to our own fears of death, or grief for someone we loved who has died. To do effective counselling we need to deal with our own fears and feelings, so that we are able to concentrate on our clients and not become upset while working.

Counselling children about other people's deaths

Sometimes caregivers may keep a death secret from a child. However, research shows it is better for children to hear about the death of someone close from someone they trust. If they are not told, and hear from someone else by accident, they may lose trust in, and feel angry with, caregivers for withholding the information.

Children under five years old may think that death is reversible. When working with them we need to use

> Session 10 is a useful resource; it contains information and exercises about understanding death, the cycle of life, and coping with loss.

simple stories and explanations. For example, first explore together whether a dead insect can walk, eat, see, breathe, and so on. You can then explain that it will never do those things again, because it is dead: it cannot come back to life. You can make this fact less sad by explaining the cycle of life: that the insect's offspring are alive; or that the insect becomes fertilizer for the next plants to grow, and for the next insects to feed on.

Children aged between five and 10 are more likely to know that death is irreversible. They may also understand that it is unavoidable and that it happens to every living thing. However, they tend to resist the idea of their own death. Compared to younger children, they are likely to be more aware of, and affected by, the possibility or actuality of the death of someone they care about.

Children over 10 years old tend to understand the long-term implications of death and the facts associated with death. They experience emotions which are similar to those experienced by adults, but may find it hard to express them.

Whatever the age of the child, we can:
- encourage them to express their emotions through drawing, playing, storytelling, writing, and talking;
- support them in dealing with their anger, guilt, fears, and worries;
- reassure them that their reactions are normal;
- bring a photo or memento to the counselling session, to bring the person who has died symbolically into the session;
- talk about the person who has died by sharing their happy memories and considering how to keep the memory of them alive;
- encourage the child and caregiver to create a memory book or box, containing items to help remember the person who is dying or who has died;
- explore any particular memory which troubles them (as people often get stuck on a certain occurrence in relation to the person's sickness or death) and help them make sense of this in its wider context;
- think about who is left to support them, and how to continue with their lives.

> In Exercise 11.6 participants identify special dates to remember people who have died.
>
> Use the jigsaw in Exercise 2.6 to support the child to take scattered troubling memories and turn them into a whole, and more positive, picture.
>
> In Exercise 10.5 children make a bracelet where each bead represents someone who cares for them.

We can also explain to the caregiver that when children want to talk about death, it is good to respond to them. Support the caregiver in explaining the situation to the child, and in being sensitive to their needs.

Counselling about a child's own death

Children may be worried about the possibility of their own death, even if they are not ill. This is particularly likely if they know a child who has died. In counselling we can:
- help children talk about their fears, and reassure them that lots of people worry about death;
- help them understand death as a fact of life, and part of the cycle of life;
- find out about their religious beliefs, and how they fit into the child's sense of agency and support;
- explain that we do not have complete control over our health, but that our actions (e.g. taking medication correctly) do have an important influence on it;

- support them in considering what they can do to increase their chance of good health, and in thinking about how to live their life.

You may also need to give support to children in the final stage of AIDS. Here are some tips about working in this situation.

- Work with caregivers and others to create a loving environment, e.g. using music that the child likes; appropriate touch such as gentle massage of the limbs; sweet-scented flowers, shells or stones; tastes that the child likes; and the presence of people whom the child loves;

- Support caregivers in coping with the situation, and in accepting that the child is dying. Explain that their acceptance makes it easier for the child to die peacefully, when it is time.

- If the child wants to talk about their approaching death, encourage them to do so.

- Answer questions about death openly, simply and honestly. If the child asks 'Am I going to die?', you might turn the question back by saying 'You have asked whether you are going to die; what do you think? What does death mean to you?'

- Encourage the child to talk about their fears and respond appropriately.

- Allow them to express sorrow, anger; do not attempt to cheer them up.

- Let the child talk about how they want to be remembered, if they want to.

- Do not give expectations of recovery; if the child or caregivers think the child will recover you can explore that, without agreeing or disagreeing with them.

- Discuss with the child their religious beliefs and, if necessary, connect them to sources of spiritual support.

Final words

We hope this guide is useful to you in your important work. It can be difficult to do our work well when there are lots of clients and not enough time, and when their stories touch us and we may feel powerless against the challenges they face. But we know that good counselling really does help adults and children. We hope you will have the courage to develop your skills in counselling children and their caregivers, and will work, with your colleagues, to raise standards for the benefit of those children and their communities.

Sources of information

Human Sciences Research Council (2012) *Legal, Ethical and Counselling Issues Related to HIV Testing of Children; HIV Counselling and Testing of Children: Implementation Guidelines*, Msunduzi, South Africa: HSRC <http://www.hsrc.ac.za/uploads/pageContent/3181/HIVc ounsellingandtestingofchildren-implementationguidelinesWEB.pdf> [accessed 14 October 2015].

Southern African AIDS Training (SAT) Programme (2003) *Guidelines for Counselling Children who are Infected with HIV or Affected by HIV and AIDS*, Harare: SAT Programme <www. k4health.org/sites/default/files/Couselling_Children.pdf> [accessed 14 October 2015].